WHY ME
Living without Conceiving
WHY NOT ME

Pamela Thomas

3G Publishing, Inc.
Loganville, Ga 30052
www.3gpublishinginc.com
Phone: 1-888-442-9637

First published by 3G Publishing, Inc. July, 2020

ISBN: 978-1-941247-79-2

Printed in the United States of America

Disclaimer: Although the author and publisher have made every effort to ensure that the information in this book was correct at press time, the author and publisher do not assume and hereby disclaim any liability to any party for any loss, damage, or disruption caused by errors or omissions, whether such errors or omissions result from negligence, accident, or any other cause. This book is not intended as a substitute for the medical advice of physicians. The reader should regularly consult a physician in matters relating to his/her health and particularly concerning any symptoms that may require diagnosis or medical attention.

Dedication

In the loving memory of my father, grandparents, and auntie Annie Mae.

Acknowledgments

Many people who have blessed my life, especially my husband, family, and friends as well as my church family.

Contents

INTRODUCTION

As I begin to write this book with tears in my eyes, I utterly understand it is all because you needed to perceive you are not alone. I realize you may have never heard of me, and that is fine because soon you will never forget me. I have been on this earth for over fifty years. This book will share my dreams, preparation for my future, my success, my pain, my anger, my purpose and much more. Before I truly get started, I must Praise God for this journey called life. Life can be challenging trying to find purpose through your pressures and pain.

Many years I have recognized my purpose is to share my story with someone as special as you. Life is not made to be easy and many times we will question God. Yes, it is okay to question God because his title is God, and he has no name because he is I AM. I am whatever you need. Many years I procrastinated and finally, enough was enough for someone needed to realize you can make it and survive. I felt and still feel the pain of young and seasoned ladies trying to bear a child or children and I began to write my story.
As I continue to evolve into the woman God

would have me to be, it blows my mind how we grow in GRACE. But in the growth, I will never forget my journey. So, relax yes, I sense that many of you think you cannot relax and there is no peace because I used to be that one. I used to say time waits on no one.

Life -- the dictionary states "it is the existence of an individual human or animal." I used to say what is my life without children, but life is different in the eyes of many. Happiness is the meaning and the purpose of life, the entire cycle from the beginning to the end of human existence.
So, come take this journey with me about my LIFE.

Chapter 1: Growing Up with a Dream

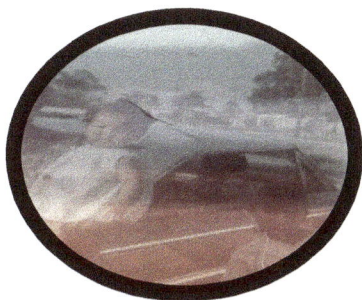

I am Pam and I grew up playing house and with dolls like so many others while watching my mother who is my best friend and my idol prepare daily for another day. Back then I did not utterly understand the meaning of a MOTHER. Watching her made it look interesting and awesome all at the same time. She was so organized and so prissy and precise. The dictionary defines a mother as a woman in relation to her child or children. A female parent, a woman in authority. The transitive verb definition is to give birth, to produce, to care for, or protect. I took comfort in knowing my mother was in control and protected me at all costs and times. I wanted to follow her and mimic her. Mother excelled as a gifted educator by day and my extraordinary mother by day/night. Although I am not the only child; I am the baby girl. However, she made me feel like I was the only child on this earth. I soon found out she enabled everybody to discover their exceptional qualities. Even to this day, her students talk about how special she was to them.

My father was a Principal but all I saw with these young eyes was my mother. A mother has a nurturing interaction that cannot be explained. She was my everything -- I must say it again. She was my protector, disciplinarian, and my friend. My mother was selfless and made so many sacrifices for her children. She was laying the foundation and developing me to BECOME. She was my role model. It was evident that she loved me with all her heart and soul.

Being her child made me want to dream. So many nights I dreamed of being a mother like her. The dictionary states a dream is a series of thoughts, images, and sensations occurring in a person's mind during sleep. It is a cherished aspiration, ambition, or ideal. In my eyes and my mind, I just indulged in daydreams and fantasied with this greatly desired thought to become a mother just like my mother.

I began to walk like her, talk like her, and treat the dolls the way she treated me. I would maintain the dolls ready for school and church. I even told the dolls that communion was required on the 1st Sunday. I told them how important Sunday school was. I taught them how to listen and follow directions. I shared with my dolls how you must not talk loudly. A lady should be seen not to be heard first. They learned how to match clothes and shoes with a purse. They learned how important it was to take baths. How to brush their teeth and to eat an important first meal of the day, which was Breakfast, and do not forget to say your grace. How to be on time and how to plan so there is no need to rush and be unorganized and not prepared. Yes, this list can go on and on.

The foundation is so important in a child's life. A foundation is what will hold you together during rough times. Parents start the book of your discovery. I was able to understand that the process of my learning ultimately began with my mom. The direction a child will go starts with a mother's love or parents' love. So, my main desire was to please my mom and to make her proud of me. She showed me how to be happy, but she also showed me how to overcome when you are sad. She prepared me for when I would apprehend yes and when I would apprehend no. Thus, I will always remember that no is not a rejection but a no (at this time) redirection. A mother is so many things and wears so many hats. Many times, in life we do not understand a mother until we get older, wiser, and become a mother ourselves.

I am so glad that God chose me for my mother. I could write another book just about her. Yes, just because of this book my next book may just be on my mother. Her teaching, actions, beliefs, nurturing and direction can take me right into my next chapter of this book -- Preparing for My Future.

Chapter 2: Preparing for My Future

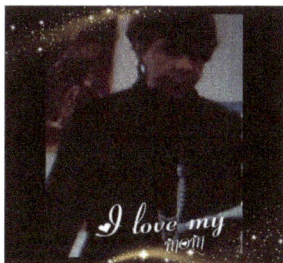

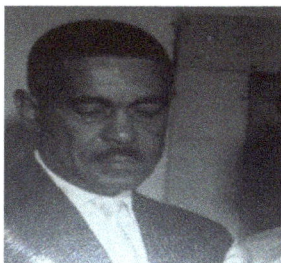

After watching my mom demonstrate what a mother looks like with grace and pride has made me eager to become a mother. Now was the time for me to use my foundation, skills, and prepare for my future. In preparing for my future, my main desire was to please my mom and myself all at the same time.

Life, in the beginning, seems easy but when you grow in wisdom you will find out quickly life is hard. So, my main goals were to complete high school and move on to college. Was achieving goals easy you may ask? No, but along the way, I learned so much and all my trials and tribulations made me who I am today. During my life, my mother demonstrated with actions on how to live and avoid conflict. The grace that my mother demonstrated I did not master until I became older with knowledge, wisdom, and experience.

I had the opportunity to enjoy all the things a little girl could encounter. From being a cheerleader, majorette, clarinet player, band member, choir member, flag twirler, college freshman queen, Psychology Major Leader, Who's Who Among Students, and much more. I just wanted to make my parents happy and my future family, children happy. I found what I truly needed at a young age to make it through and that BEST thing was the belief in GOD. I had some dark days which will be in my future book; but with God, I was able to survive and come out on top.

When I was young my mother and father took me all over the world. I realize I do not remember much. My father was a busybody so after him being a principal during the week he just wanted to travel on the weekends and the summer and every holiday. My mom was a teacher and the mother of three. I was even blessed to have a nanny. Yes, I was the baby and 10 years apart from my middle sister. I always felt like I was the only one because I enjoyed being the baby and alone for a very long time. All this time together continued to allow me to dream of becoming a mother. I wanted the same things I saw and was allotted. Things like a family, an education, houses, cars, and the freedom to be.

In the beginning, I did not understand paying bills, getting up daily to make it to work, and all the responsibilities that come with being an adult. So, I innocently enjoyed the ride and dreamed.

As a little girl, I can remember dreaming of the big house on the hill with three children running around, and a working husband. I could see myself in a career and being a good wife and mother. I wanted to be able to cook, clean, and boss the family but at the same time submit to a husband.

I would imagine waking up my family to the aromas of a traditional southern breakfast wafting and swirling throughout the house announcing that Sunday breakfast of bacon, cheese grits, toast, pancakes, and sausage is ready for prayer and consumption and then off to Sunday school and church. In my mind on Sundays we would always have to be there on the 1st Sunday for communion. Communion was the service of Christian Worship at which bread and wine are consecrated and shared. The Lord's Supper was to commemorate the death of Christ. The elements used to represent Christ's body and blood are bread and wine. I remember we always did a confession. Back then I may not have understood everything in its entirety, but confessions were required in my home and confessions would be required in my future home.

The foundation was strong with both actions and words. So, I continued to move with a plan. I completed high school and went on to college. I completed my undergrad in Psychology and moved to the big city of Atlanta, Georgia. I started looking for a job which was not easy. I worked as a teacher, counselor, and manager in retail. I worked at Equifax to be able to understand credit better and then I landed my dream job at General Electric, which changed my life. My dreams were coming true and lining up with my plan. I met the love of my life. I went back to school and received my MBA, and I decided to go back again and receive another master's in human resource management.

I was attending a great church and my mom was proud of her baby girl. I was growing in so many areas. I was setting goals and reaching them all as planned. I was determined to make my mom proud and be happy at the same time. Life is not as easy as many pretend it is but keep on living and you will see for yourself. There will be times in your life where you will have to make decisions that will affect your future. You will have to go with your intuition, which is your gut feelings.

During this time in your life, you must be careful who you are connected to as they could make you or break you. Will you make some mistakes? This might be your question, and you sure may or may not, but no one is perfect? I would always remember an old saying that with every choice you make there is a consequence. I would recommend that you learn from all mistakes – let mistakes be a teachable moment. Planning for your future is not easy when in that stage in life it is difficult to comprehend who you really are

Chapter 3: Getting Married

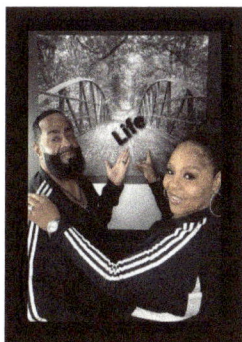

The bible defines marriage as a covenant. God sketched his original plan for marriage in when man (Adam) and one woman (Eve) united to become one flesh. In Genesis 2:24 (The English Standard Version), it says that "Therefore a man shall leave his father and mother and hold fast to his wife, and they shall become one flesh." I have always taken marriage seriously. I had been engaged before, and I am so glad the doors were closed. Therefore, I always say rejection is not bad, but it is a form of redirection. I thank God for all the closed doors. I took the time to focus on self and allow God to help prepare me for the husband he had for me. I enjoyed loving myself and the pruning stage.

When I first met my future husband, I knew the Lord had smiled down on me. He was indeed something to look at. I praise God for favor. Yes, I realize that in Proverbs 18:22 (The King James Version),it says "Whoso findeth a wife findeth a good thing, and obtained favor of the Lord" but I received some favor too. This man captured my attention so easily. In the beginning, I had my guard and walls up because I did not want to be hurt again. But I enjoyed his conversation, his respect for women, his kind heart, his gentleness, his style, his walk, his smile, and of course his bad boy side.

When you allow God to control the situation you cannot and will not go wrong. God was smiling down on me by saying you did the right thing by bowing down to me and I answered your prayers. I slowly but surely fell in love with this wonderful man. You must pray and move out of the way totally to receive what God has for you. The bible said, and I must repeat, that when a man finds a wife, he finds a good thing and obtains favor from the Lord. My dreams were truly coming to pass. After two years of dating, he proposed to me and I became his wife. Like so many other women I dreamed of that one day, and oh, what a day. That was one day I will never forget. I had a beautiful wedding with a huge wedding party, the church was filled with my family and friends and so much love was in the room. We had tears and peace in the atmosphere. Yes, God was in the room. At the altar we formed a cross standing with my husband, myself, and God. I believed with everything in me this man was a gift from God. No, he was not all I had dreamed of or wanted, but he was all I needed. The new life for us began. We communicated and planned out our lives. One thing happened before we got married his number one lady died. This special lady was his grandmother. She had spoiled him but at the same time raised an awesome man.

When his grandmother died, the transition was like she was passing him on to the angel that was to be his wife. My God, when God is in the plan signs and wonders will line up and obtain your attention at all costs. I was so glad I had to back up and move out of God's way. I felt the grace and love God had for me through this man. God answered all my prayers and the results were like a fairy tale. Being in love is a beautiful thing for I was no longer lonely. This man became my best friend, my protector, the head of our home, and much more. He was so gentle and tenderhearted to me and knew how to handle me, which is not easy yes, I understand me. Our love for each other grew so strong and continues to grow. We laugh together, we cry together, we travel, we dream and to sum it up we just enjoy each other's company. I can write a book just about my man.

What I love about him is that he understands that we are not perfect individuals, but we are perfect for each other. He pushes me to go after my dreams. He is a humble but firm man with a gentle spirit. This union is very strong and indeed ordained by God. Many people ask me did you write down what you wanted your husband to be, and I answered I sure did but that was not what God wanted. So, God did not give me what I wanted he gave me what I needed. This is one of the reasons we have been together for over 23 years. "Therefore what God has joined together, let no one separate" (Mark 10:9, New International Version). We have agreed from day one to keep God first. We have been sowing seeds into each other since day one and this has flourished life for us today and tomorrow. When we got married, I was 29 years old. We were enjoying our careers, traveling, building our home, and so much more. Then around age 32, we started to discuss having children. Let us move forward to demonstrate some of the storms and sunshine we endured.

Chapter 4: Trying to Conceive

The conversation begins -- Honey, are you ready to have children? Since we are in a place where we can give our children all they need, and we are in a great place in our marriage the answer was YES. With excitement and determination, the Fun begins. As women, we all recognize we have a monthly cycle that usually comes every 28 days. Well, in my world being irregular my cycle would fall between 28-31 days. A woman can only become pregnant during ovulation. Ovulation is the release of eggs from the ovaries. In humans, this event occurs when the ovarian follicles rupture and release the secondary oocyte ovarian cells. After ovulation, during the luteal phase, the egg will be available to be fertilized by sperm. In this cycle, pregnancy is only possible during the five days before ovulation through to the day of ovulation. Like I stated earlier you have a 28 days' cycle, you ovulate around day 14 and your most fertile days are days 12, 13, and 14. Outside of that window the probability of pregnancy declines. Many women forget to count the days, but some women have signs to be able to recognize the feeling in their reproductive system. Research tells us that there are many signs that a woman may encounter like: mild pelvic or lower abdominal pain, sore breast, light spotting or discharge, changes in the cervix, and much more.

Trying to conceive is fun because although you realize you can only conceive during a certain time you desire to just have sex recognizing you are trying to bring in a new life into the world. During the beginning phase, we had so much fun. We laughed, we acted silly, we dreamed aloud, and we entertained the thought of having more than one child. We had sex more than the norm and norms are different for everyone. Sex was so exciting because we knew the plan was to conceive a baby girl or a baby boy, and we even did not mind having twins. Each month I would receive a little excitement because I started taking a great multivitamin from a health food store and my cycle was like clockwork. My cycle was no longer irregular my cycle would come on every 28 days. But month after month, I would become slightly more disheartened.

After about two years of marriage, my husband was rushed to the ER. He slipped in the freezer at work and continued to work with discomfort. Later that evening he encountered swelling of the scrotum with severe pain. Come to find out he had to have emergency surgery due to his testicles being twisted. Testicular torsion happens when a spermatic cord becomes twisted, cutting off the flow of the blood to the attached testicle. Most cases of testicular torsion affect guys who have a condition called a bell clapper deformity. In most males, the testicles are attached to the scrotum, making testicles hard for them to twist. During this surgery, the doctor made a small cut in the scrotum and untwisted the spermatic cord if necessary and stitch one or both testicles to the inside of the scrotum.

Surgery was a success, but the doctor asked us did we have children, and we stated we were trying to conceive. He informs us to keep trying because this could affect conception. This was a sad moment, but I was happy my husband was doing well. We tried not to think too much about this issue, but as a woman, we over-think everything. I begin to allow myself to worry in silence. I tried not to stress much because stress can also hinder conception. I started looking back over my life and I began to blame myself because I had never been pregnant before, and I was a little on the juicy/ thick side. I quickly ignored that thought because I was also on birth control pills during those times. After my husband healed, we begin to start back enjoying trying to conceive. Many couples that were married around the same time were conceiving, so you know my mind began to play tricks on me. We begin to pray more and have sex more. Yes, you can only become pregnant during a certain time, but we enjoyed the trying phase of no ovulation. We continued living and not to concern ourselves much for another two years, and, yes, time does pass by fast when you are having fun.

Eventually, I found myself moving mentally into a dark place because I was ministering to a lot of couples that were trying to conceive. Many people cannot handle these times alone and for some, I was the chosen one to help them win through these times. So, during this time I shared with my husband that I was going to investigate my insurance to see if they cover infertility.

Chapter 5: Fertility Assistance

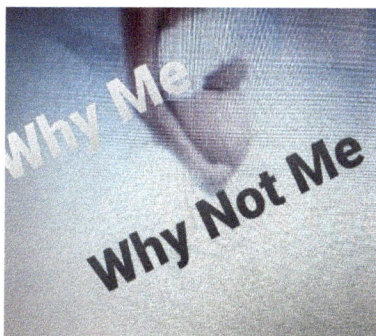

This is an uncomfortable conversation to have in a great marriage ordained by God. Being a believer and loving God with my whole heart a particular Bible verse was always coming in my thoughts. In Genesis 1:28 (The King James Version), it says that "And God blessed them, and God said unto them, Be fruitful, and multiply, and replenish the earth, and subdue it: and have dominion over the fish of the sea, and over the fowl of the air, and over every living thing that moveth upon the earth." After thinking and meditating on this verse, the reading causes sadness and questions. But let the process begin. Many of us do not even want to think about needing help to conceive but, we must be honest with self even during heartache and despondency and seek the help needed.

So, let the story commence. I decided to research and not just go by what I knew. First, let us understand that infertility is the inability to conceive a child after a certain period and for everyone the length of which varies. The term can also refer to women who are unable to carry a pregnancy to term. Infertility has multitudinous causes, including polycystic ovary syndrome and low sperm quality. I can say that the serious issue of infertility is one of the most sensitive subjects to talk about. Many people have a natural desire or a dream for fatherhood and motherhood. Many people who fall in this category have friends with no difficulties having children, but when it comes down to it you expect your experience to be no different.

After doing a lot of research, I found out that statistics show approximately one out of six couples face fertility problems. But it also has been proven that eventually, many couples do go on to have children, with or without the aid of treatments such as IVF. Times have brought on a change with medical advances offering new hope on the horizon for those facing this stressful challenge. It is sad to say that many types of treatments cost a small fortune and end in failure where some end with success.

There are many causes of infertility. Let us cover a few issues with the ovulation process. The exact nature of the issue varies between women. Sometimes no egg release occurs during the menstrual cycle, or perhaps the egg release happens in some menstrual cycles but not in others. There are several reasons this happens. For example, an overactive thyroid gland might cause ovulation problems. Also, a condition called premature ovarian failure where the ovaries cease functioning before a woman gets into her 40s. Another reason is poor quality eggs. The quality of the eggs the woman produces also affects the chances of parenthood. Many factors have a negative impact on egg health. The woman has a genetic problem in some instances, but controllable elements such as lifestyle and environment are very important influences. Women who smoke, live in polluted environments, and lead sedentary lives have lower quality, less fertile eggs. Additional factors that damage egg health include hormones and a poor-quality diet.

Another major factor of concern to many people is that fertility naturally declines with age. It has been revealed that women today try to start families at an older age. But when we were younger, we were informed to have children young like in your 30s. While social changes lead couples to postpone childbearing, how the passage of years affects the woman's biological clock remains unchanged. For some couples, the age they try to start a family will not be the issue, but the later they start the greater the prospect of infertility problems. Where sometimes there is no reason, or the reason cannot be found.

Additionally, the side effects of drugs you consume may cause fertility problems, which is part of the price abusers of narcotics often must pay. These issues also may occur with people who use prescription medications. Sometimes the interruption to fertility ceases a short while after stopping the medicine. Even prolonged use of conventional medication like painkillers or blood-thinners may harm fertility. Certain medical and surgical procedures may harm fertility. There is so much that can harm the body and cause fertility issues we may never notice, understand, or find out. As I was reading and researching, I read that several medical and surgical procedures may give rise to fertility issues. Many people have chemotherapy that causes ovarian failure, and the damage and scarring pelvic and cervical surgery may cause. All these medicines or procedures should be discussed with your health provider.

Women must realize men have fertility issues as well. We must all make sure we have our partner checked for fertility issues. After I and my husband completed so many tests all the tests showed both parties to be healthy and able to conceive only identified a tilted uterus and slow sperm count. The first thing we tried was mediation and to identify I had many follicles I produced monthly. Each month I was able to produce follicles. We never decided to freeze any for later. My husband took vitamins and made sure underwear/boxers were not tight. So, we moved to IVF (In Vitro Fertilization). This is a process where extracting eggs and gathering sperm and then manually combining the egg and sperm in a laboratory dish. The embryo or embryos are then transferred to the uterus.

There are 5 steps -1st fertility medication will be prescribed to stimulate egg production 2nd Eggs are retrieved through a minor procedure that uses ultrasound imaging to guide a hollow needle through the pelvic cavity to remove the eggs, 3rd the male sperm is then provided so it can be prepared for combining with the eggs. 4th Insemination which is the eggs and sperm are put together and stored in a laboratory dish to encourage fertilization. The eggs are monitored to confirm fertilization and cell division are taking place. Once this happens, they are considered embryos. 5th The embryos are transferred into the women's uterus three to five days following egg retrieval and fertilization. A catheter or small tube is inserted into the uterus to transfer the embryos. If the procedure is successful, implantation usually occurs around six to ten days following egg retrieval. There are a few minor side effects of IVF.

We went through this process twice with no luck. This is very hard on a couple mentally, physically, and emotionally. But it is indeed recommended because some couples have great success and you might be that one.

Chapter 6: Waiting and Praying

This was a dark place for me. Being a Christian and crying out to God for myself and others is hard to explain. During this time of my life, I was speechless at times and this dark place was indeed a test for me and my husband. Many couples were placed in my life for counseling and prayer for conception. What a TEST! Yes, wow what a TEST! But with my whole heart, I prayed and counseled others while being sad, tested, unsure, mad, disappointed, and questioning many beliefs.

Here is a testimony from a wonderful couple Donna and Jeff:

It was Summer 1998 and I and my little Girly had made the leap of faith to leave Charlotte and move to Atlanta. I had a great job, and a nice place to live, but I was scared. We did not have any family here and I was very leery about putting Girly in a daycare, but I was trusting God.

When we finally got all moved and settled in, we were missing something, a church home. At my new job

I heard several people talking about New Birth and what a wonderful church it was. I knew if I found us a good church, things would then be much better. We visited for the first time on a Wednesday, but by the time we parked and walked 20 minutes to the church, we were late. I was tired from work, but Girly and I had the best time. In the end, we both said let us come back Sunday. We met some amazing people and loved our church. One beautiful lady just stood out to me. She was gorgeous, always smiling, and Girly loved being near her. Her name was Pam.

We visited for a couple of months and then we joined. In the midst of all this God had sent MY HIM. It was like a fairy tale, and I just could not believe this was all happening to me. We got engaged and decided to get married on 1/1/2000. Soon after we got married, we decided to start having children. He was 30 and I was 29, so we did not want to waste time. Unfortunately, when we went in for our pre-preconception checkup my gynecologist said she had found a grapefruit-sized cyst on one of my ovaries and it had to be removed right away. She then told us more devastating news that by removing one of my ovaries our chances of getting pregnant would be reduced by half. I was distraught and felt after all these blessings WHY ME? I went in for the surgery and when I woke up my husband Jeff, my Mommy, and my gynecologist were all looking at me as if

I had won a prize. Finally, my gynecologist burst out I SAVED YOUR OVARY! I started crying and thanking God. We were told we had to start trying right away to increase our chances. I told Pam and she said they were trying too. We were so happy. Every month my cycle came I went into depression, but Pam seemed fine and still believing as strong as ever. Finally, a year later we got pregnant with fertility treatment and God. I was nervous about telling Pam because I loved her so much and did not want to hurt her. I waited for a while and finally, I told her. She had the biggest smile on her face and hugged me so tight I could feel her love come through me. It took 8 long years to have our family, and Pam was right there loving me all along the way. She never once showed an ounce of jealousy.

Pam never really seemed depressed like I had been, but I was not in her private place with God. I remember her telling me something like do not feel bad for me, be the best Mommy you can be. How on earth could she really feel that way? Wasn't she robbed, hurt, disappointed, and mad?

Twenty years have passed now, and Pam never did have a biological child. But God had a plan. A beautiful plan. A beautiful baby girl was born, and her parents were not able to care for her the way she needed. You guessed it, Pam and her husband could!

They have a beautiful daughter and she is their perfect gift from God. There are so many more things that happened over these 20 years, but the most important of all was that God sent two women to share a journey, and we BOTH learned what he wanted us to know.

I love you Pam, and your love and friendship have changed my life forever!

Yes, I counsel people; it is my calling. With a degree in Psychology, I was able to become a counselor after college. I did not stay in that field long, but it was and will be a part of my life for the rest of my life. My ministry is to the lost, hurting and those that lack guidance. My undying passion is to lead people by example and help them gain clarity in their expectations. Through determination and unwavering faith, this goal is achievable. I am inclined to support, guide, and serve the needs of others. I have committed myself to walk people through the process. I find myself specializing in married couples, teens, and whoever God laid on my heart to help. Everyone is not for you to help, but God knows who is. I help people instead of direct people. I have the trust of people. I speak in love. I build people up. I provide clear and obtainable expectations. I am always available with God's direction. I am honest, and

I am the one who cares for people. I have learned that my MOTIVATION IS NOT SIMPLY PEOPLE, BUT THEIR GROWTH, WELL-BEING, AND OVERALL LIFE JOURNEY.

Fear was consuming my mind and body. The stress was unbearable, and I was praying on the level of my faith. I always believed my greatest weapon was my prayer life. I was beginning to ask God for the strength to endure. I was asking and crying for direction, peace, and understanding. I acknowledged I had a gift to help other people but during this time of my life, it seemed like I could not help myself. I cried and I prayed, and I stood as still as I could, and nothing was working. I was questioning God. Yes, I said it, I did question God. God already knew I would question him for he is all-knowing.

Sadness is a dark, lonely place and takes a strong person to handle these moments without going into depression. With Psychology being my undergrad major, because I understand the different stages a person can go through, I was able to not feel but see myself headed in the wrong direction. I was crying out to the one that had kept me for years, the one that never left me, and the one that would answer all my prayers. He did not answer them all when I wanted them answered, but he was always on time; and the ones he did not answer he would show me in a dream, or right in my face. In my life I have dreams and many of my dreams have come true. So, I was waiting for a dream so I could receive a better understanding or direction. During this time in my life, I was saying what did I do wrong to deserve this. I reminded God of his words again "And God blessed them, and God said unto them, Be fruitful, and multiply, and replenish the earth, and subdue it: and have dominion over the fish of the sea, and over the fowl of the air, and over every living thing that moveth upon the earth." These were not my words but God's words.

Life got worse before it got better. Being able to reach out to others like my mom and close friends helped me deal with guilt and anger. I was also informed during this time that couples experiencing psychological stress had poorer results with infertility treatment. Believe me, I tried hard to reduce stress in my life before trying to become pregnant, and during the process, but words are easier said than done. I am a true believer, so I would remind myself that the Bible states in Philippians 4:6-8 (The New International Version) "Do not be anxious about anything, but in everything by prayer and supplication with thanksgiving let your requests be made known to

God. And the peace of God, which surpasses all understanding, will guard your hearts and your minds in Christ Jesus. Finally, brothers, whatever is true, whatever is honorable, whatever is just, whatever is pure, whatever is lovely, whatever is commendable, if there is any excellence, if there is anything worthy of praise, think about these things." The more I quoted the Word the unhappier I became.

Can you believe that everyone I was praying for got pregnant except for me? CAN YOU BELIEVE THIS? Pregnancy happened, and I was happy for them and thank God for answering the prayers of me and others. On the other hand, can you imagine how I felt? I will tell you just how I felt -- sad, unsure, unclear, let down, disappointed, sorrowful, rejected, dejected, miserable, downhearted, regretful, low-spirited, broken and brokenhearted, gloomy, joyless, and even MAD. After a few weeks or maybe months, I was still shaken and not at ease. I continued to press on but to tell the truth, it was hard to pray after the prayers for others were answered. Again, I cried out to God, WHY ME? He probably was answering me, but I was not in the place to hear.

I continued to pray with tears in my eyes. I was young and had not been married long, and we were building together so many would say why did not you acquire a surrogate. Do you realize the cost of a surrogate? Also, during those times surrogacy was not talked much about. Here I go thinking about maybe I am too large and that is one of the causes of infertility, but then, around the time of my thinking a heavy-set woman would walk by looking nine months pregnant. Here I go in my feelings again so imagine my thoughts. Yes, whatever you thought I probably thought twice. I was so tired of crying and thinking. I am truly an over-thinker. By this time, I had no more faith and I was angry.

Chapter 7: Being Angry

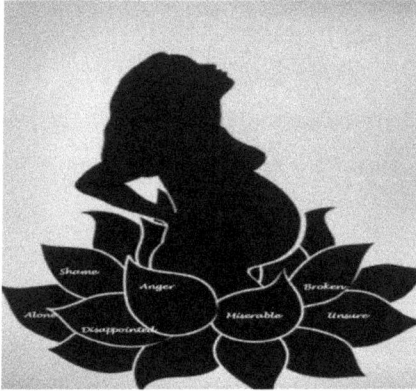

Being angry is so draining, miserable, and dark.
The dictionary defines angry as filled with anger,
having a strong feeling of being upset or annoyed,
and showing anger. This place and time in my life
was very dark with so many unpleasant thoughts
entering my mind. Being angry can cause many
problems like becoming sick, trigger physiological
reactions, and can also have long-term effects on
the body. Anger can identify as so bad that you
can have a cardiac arrest, fainting spells, stroke,
high blood pressure, and mental conditions. People
around you can notice or discern your pain. I do
believe that hurt people really do hurt people.

Because if you are not mindful you can cause emotional and psychological damage to family and friends. Anger is often associated with negative connotations. Yet, anger is not all bad. Some of the most successful people I have personally met have little to no reservations about unleashing their anger. There is management and how to harness the power of it. Everybody experiences some type of anger and many feel embarrassed and even ashamed whenever they display anger.

While being angry, it is important to understand that anger is not all bad. There are good elements to being angry as well. To me, I would rather be perceived as angry than depressed. I noticed most people would accommodate those who are angry. During this time, I realized you become in-the-moment. That moment in time took me to a place I had never been mentally before. I could not control my thoughts, my actions, my words, or my temper. This place was dark and lonely. I did not like the emotions of hopelessness and despair in this place. It took a toll on me in that still place. This is one of the reasons I am writing this book, to be able to help one person is my heart's desire.

I was so mad that I was asking God "why me, why me, why me?" The one who speaks, lives and breathes your name. The one who chose to do right when I could have done wrong. Fascinating how this appears to happen a lot, how good people seem to be punished constantly. I was sick and tired of being sick and tired. In life, it always seems that good people either die or to befall sickness. I have always questioned this in life. During this time, I found myself listening to sad music and watching crazy and sad TV shows. Life sometimes makes the situation so easy to fall in the trap of enough is enough. This is one reason why people may commit suicide, etc.

I pray any thought of self-destruction to be removed from your mind and heart because you are somebody and this is only a phase you are going through. That dark place was a difficult place to pull myself out of and that place is truly a deep miserable funk, but I had to find a way to accept and conquer this disappointment. This disappointment I do not wish on anyone reading this book. I pray God releases peace that covers your mind and heart and gives you directions to overcome. You will be able to accept and conquer this moment in time. Times like these may be hard, but you are not alone. Many people may be going through this or have gone through it. Just hold on and you will be okay, for you have a destiny and a purpose for your life. Someone truly does need you to survive.

Chapter 8: Accepting and Conquering

My father's mother passed when he was an infant. I began to do research on her death because one night I had a dream of passing while giving birth. So, the only thing that came to mind was the death of my grandmother whom I never knew. My searching was getting nowhere, and my siblings did not have much information. I begin searching a little harder and the spirit told me no need to search.

The thought of me passing giving birth caught me at a loss for words. As much as I was hoping, wishing, praying, crying, and angry, sadly none of those feelings compared to the thought of death. My reading and research revealed that about 700 women die each year in the United States because of pregnancy or delivery complications. I thought of the possibility I could have been in that number Lord. So, my mind started to shift into being in a thankful mode. I started to become thankful and accepting the love God genuinely does have for me, and I successfully started to overcome all my fears. Accepting and knowing are two different things with a great reward. As bad as I wanted to bring a life into the world, I did not want to spare my life in the process. Many great women did die giving birth. Oh, what a day when life begins to flash in front of your eyes. Imagine delivering a healthy baby and losing the mother. I do understand death happens every day and God has a reason. I truly did not want my family to have to carry this for the rest of their lives because of something we desired. Many great families deal with this and have great stories to share and some may not. I did not understand during this time of my life how great my calling was on this earth. Now I understand I had to change and save some lives.

God had a plan for my life that outweighed my desire at the time. God is always leading us somewhere, and we do not always understand what is happening during those times. But no matter what is going on in your life everything is the way it is for a reason. I simply did not have the faith, but I recognize my life was his plan. When God takes something from you or does not give you something, he is not punishing you but merely opening you up to receive something better. I can say today that the Will of God will never take you where the Grace of God will not protect you and your mind. I had to start totally trusting God and to understand my strength is in him. I could not conquer the peace that passes all understanding until I laid prostrate at his feet empty. I was running from the presence of God, but God was never running from me. He was right there all the time. I was told so many times in the past that all things work together for the good of them who loves the Lord, but I had to walk life out to understand that scripture. Walking in your belief and/or unbelief is not a smooth walk in the park. Some days I felt like I was drowning, and no life jacket was in sight.

I started to see light at the end of the tunnel. During this time, I was still seeing the fertility specialist and getting a lot of results back. My head was starting to be in the right place. So, when receiving feedback my attitude and tone had shifted. The doctors and nurses were so applauding of my responses that they stated I needed to come to speak when they had meetings with families going through infertility issues in life. They said I need to travel and speak on the subject. Little did I perceive that God was preparing me to write and share my story with you. Everyone's story will not end the same. Many people will succeed with treatments and many will not. Some will be able to afford a surrogate, and some will not. Some will have multiple children, and some will have miscarriages. Others the doctor will find nothing major wrong with the female and something wrong with the male. But God already wrote the story we are living.

Many would say I should have done more, and I say enough is enough. What God has for me is for me and what he does not have for me is just not for me. I started to focus on myself and how to become a better me and search to see what I had that could help others. During this time God continued to place so many people in my path who needed my help to become who God ordained them to become. I ran long enough, and I am still running a bit because I am human, and I am very hard on myself. So, I asked God "WHY ME?" What do I have that lures people to me, and I end up helping them? God would always remind me I have already placed in you what you need for who you are to touch in life. It is so important for us to line up with God's calling because someone is waiting for us to be in place. Everything began to fall in place and one chapter ended in my life and a new chapter started.

Chapter 9: Adopting in the Midst of It All

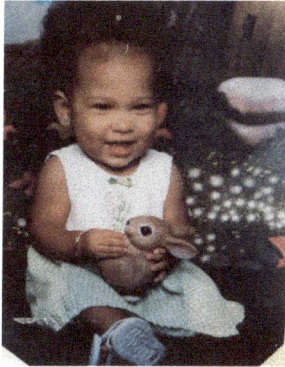

Oh, my God, who would have ever imagined this road. This path was a road I was placed on seemingly like in a blink of an eye. When life has or is dragging you with difficulties and unanswered prayers, life is redirecting you into something great. I just had to stay focused and survive the storm. The storm took me into a direction I would have never imagined or even asked for.

During the peaceful moment in my married life and an unfamiliar time with sickness with my grandmother and great aunt, a situation happened in the family that we were not accustomed to or familiar with. A little angel was placed in the foster care system. My aunt and grandmother made a request clear that someone in the family needs to step up and make sure we took care of this issue. The issue was not a familiar one, but the request was a child that was our family. So, when my husband and I were approached, we went into prayer and God ordered our steps and directed our path. Through all the different processes and procedures, we eventually adopted our Angel.

Our child was not formed under my heart but in my heart. I promised God that I would do everything I could to raise her to be the best and that she would understand who she was and whose she was. I taught her to pray daily. I realized that no matter what the situation was or how the situation happened the plan was indeed according to God's will. No matter what we go through in life and when we do not understand, God has and is working everything out. This angel has been a blessing in our lives, and we have blessed her all in one. My great-niece became my daughter. I taught her from a baby to pray daily for her biological parents because God chose them to bring this life into the world. I praise him daily because I am not one hundred percent sure if I would have lived or died bringing a child into the world. God chose me to nurture and raise this chosen vessel. My goal is for God to say well done my good and faithful servant.

Adoption has so many positive advantages like raising a child, fulling dreams, adding joy and laughter to your home, and so much more. But you must be ready for the distresses that may surface like the mental state or emotional health that a child may go through. You must make sure to understand self-esteem and identity issues. The child will have many questions and be unsure about many things. All of this is important, and you must make sure gaining this responsibility is the most or best possible choice made with love, understanding, patience, and peace. I tell numerous people there are so many children in the system who are all alone, and they really do need you or a family to love and be loved in return. My husband is the best and hardest father I have seen. He loves this angel with his whole heart. He wants the best for her in every area of her life. He is always there for her, and he affirms he promises to be the real father he never had. He will be there mentally, physically, emotionally, spiritually, and financially. He has done just that and more.

There is no book on how to be a parent. You must do your best and provide all that you can provide. The way you think is a high percentage of the way you live. We share with so many teenagers and adults that a person can only give what they have. I remind myself and my family that everything in life is about priorities. What you prioritize will dictate what your life looks like. This child is our priority and everything that comes along with her. The how, when, and where no longer matters to me. The now is worth it all. Seeing her laugh, smile, speak her first words, take her first steps, dance, play, cheer, read, write, cry, pray, talk-back, think she senses everything, study, learn to drive, graduate, go to college, first date and all were worth my tears and heartache from not conceiving a child. This book was written in love, and I will wrap this phase up in my last chapter.

Chapter 10: Writing the BOOK and Releasing It All after 50 Years of Age Especially for YOU

Every chapter of my life I shared with you in this book was worth every moment. Life has formed me into who I am today. The unfamiliar pain that gripped me deep from within helped produce my purpose. There were nights I cried until I could not cry anymore because of reasons that were hidden and undiscoverable when I wanted them to be present. Perhaps it was the loneliness when I was surrounded by people and/or the anger I did not even realize was instilled in me that led to the heartache of questioning God, "WHY ME?"

There was silence when I needed a word accompanied by directions and paths that were too dark to explain. The voices that I studied in college and helped others to overcome seem to run me crazy. Some days the mountains were too high and too steep for me to climb, and the past happy moments were too far away for me to enjoy. I longed for the children playing that I could not call my own. And, ultimately, the sadness of trying to conceive and receiving no exciting news. What a chapter in my life that I never thought would end. God knew one day I had to write this book to help you understand that pain does not last always. Many of these chapters of my story may be your yesterday or today but let me share what your tomorrow may look like. I needed to remind you that God has a plan; and if you do not see the reason before you leave this earth, the plan still will be manifested. I can honestly say I understand your pain. I understand your anger. I understand your tears. Do not give up or give in.

Do I understand the entire plan? No, but I am at peace because God chose me to raise his angel and I gracefully accept his plan. She had a reason to be on this earth, and I was a part of God's plan. I gave her back to God the day he gave her to me with a promise to do my best in raising her to BE. So, I have an answer now why me because he could trust me. I passed his test when I did not see the way. I passed the test in the darkest time of my life, but he turned on a light when the time was right. The quieter I became the more I was able to hear. I will always remember the plan is not my will but God's will.

Many people will see the outer shell of you, but God sees and knows the inner chambers of your heart. So, remember you can survive even when times seem dark and lonely. Why me, why me, why me was the question but all the time God was saying why not you. You were chosen for this life when you were born. I accept my why not me. I am one person that may have thought I was going through hell, but I walked out of the flames carrying all my tears full of water for many like you that may be consumed by the fire.

My prayer is to help one person with this book and that one just might be you. This aspiration is paramount in the sharing of my story with you. Conception is a gift many people experience. Those of us who do not experience the gift should find a way to accept and move on. Admittedly, there will be dark times, but my prayer is that you allowed me to be your Beacon of light to usher you to your open blessings. Why you, why not you. Now is your time to help someone else. Please reach out and share this book or what you have learned with others. Even if only one word changed your life, remember that one word may be all you needed to change everything. Yes, someone needs to hear from YOU too.

Why Me, Why Not me or YOU!

REFERENCES

Medically reviewed by Deborah Weatherspoon, Ph.D., R.N., CRNA -- Written by Danielle Dresden https://www.medicalnewstoday.com/articles/324829 on March 29, 2019

Medically reviewed by Holly Ernst, PA-C -- Written by Julie Marks -- Updated on March 7, 2019, https://www.healthline.com/health/womens-health/spotting-before-periods

Urology Care Foundation. The official Foundation of the American Urological Association. What is Testicular Torsion? https://www.urologyhealth.org/urologic-conditions/testicular-torsion Retrieved December 2019

© 1998-2020 Mayo Foundation for Medical Education and Research (MFMER). All rights reserved. Infertility https://www.mayoclinic.org/diseases-conditions/infertility/symptoms-causes/syc-20354317

© 1993-2020 Reproductive Partners. Lifestyle and Fertility. https://www.reproductivepartners.com/lifestyle-fertility.html

Jun 22, 2018, 12:58:53 PM / by Center of Reproductive Medicine What is In Vitro Fertilization (IVF)? https://www.infertilitytexas.com/blog/what-is-in-vitro-fertilization-ivf

ABOUT THE AUTHOR

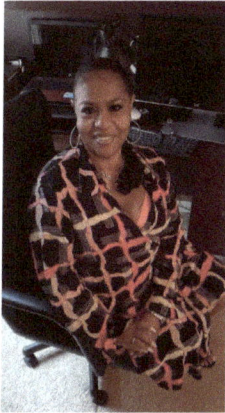

Meet Pamela Thomas, BA, MBA, MHRM, and AVP in Corporate America. I am a Child of GOD, Wife, Mother, and Author, Trainer, Speaker, Ministerial Life/Marriage Counselor. One of my goals is to teach couples how to stay together during the storm and after the storm. I coach women and teens on how to be the best version of themselves and how to align that with God's purpose for their lives. As a Purpose Engineer and Counselor, I am the visionary of ITSALLABOUTYOUTOOWITHTEARS.

My mission is to equip people with the armor needed to be all they were placed on this earth to be and to be successful personally, spiritually, and professionally for we all are important. I genuinely believe there is a link between what your passion is and what your purpose is. If you just take a few moments to think about an area of your passion and one incident that caused you great pain, I promise you that you will discover how you were able to overcome the pain -- this can birth your true purpose.

I am the owner of ITSALLABOUTYOUVIP where I am an extraordinary Consultant, Director, and Event Planner Coordinator specializing in wedding, receptions, parties, and dinner; and the Co-Owner of P & P Cakes, Sweets and Treats, where all items remind you of your grandmother's old-fashioned, home-styled sweets.

www.ingramcontent.com/pod-product-compliance
Lightning Source LLC
Chambersburg PA
CBHW051432270326
41934CB00018B/3484